Call Center Training and Ethics for Professionals

Written by Rev. Dr. Kevin T. Coughlin Ph.D.

This book is a work of nonfiction.

First Printing

Copyright © 2017 Rev. Dr. Kevin T. Coughlin Ph.D.

KTC Publishing Phase IIC Coaching, LLC

All Rights Reserved.

As permitted under the US Copyright Act of 1976, no part of this publication may be reproduced, distributed, or transmitted in any form or by any means (electronic, mechanical, photocopying, recording, or otherwise, stored in a database or retrieval system, without prior written permission of the copyright holder of this book, except by a reviewer, who may quote brief passages in a review.

The scanning, uploading, and distribution of this book via the Internet or other means without the written permission of the copyright holder and publisher is illegal and punishable by law. Please purchase only authorized electronic editions, and do not participate in or encourage electronic piracy of copyrighted materials. Your support of the author is appreciated.

Printed in the United States of America

ISBN 978-1976147654 (paperback)

Table of Contents

Description 4
Call Center Agent Training 6
Agent Responsibility 8
Becoming an Excellent Call Center Agent 9
New Laws and Landscape in Treatment 10
Problem-Solving 101 11
Active Listening is the greatest Communication Tool Agents Have! 12
Ethics 13
Code of Ethical Conduct 14
Call Center Training with Scripts 17
80/20 Rule 20
Clarify Expectations of Treatment: 21
Making Sure Clients Get the Correct level of Care 22
Referral, Engagement, and Assessment: 23
Addiction and Treatment 25
Admissions Procedure Manual: 26
The Art of Closing a Deal 29
The Psychological Reasons People Make Decisions 31
Closing Deals 33
Twelve Closing Phrases that Make Deals Happen 39
It's All About the Clients! 40
Definitions 41
Rev. Dr. Kevin T. Coughlin Ph.D. Publication Credits 54
About the Author 59
Follow Rev. Kev. on Social Media 60

Description

Call Center Training and Ethics for professionals is a book that all professionals working in the treatment industry should read. The priority of successful facilities is saving lives! The goal for detox units, residential treatment centers, PHPs, IOPs, halfway houses, or sober living facilities is to fill their empty beds with quality clients that need their services. Ethics mandate that clients be matched with the facility that can best meet their needs. Many facilities struggle to maintain their census with the proper clients for their facility. Owners and managers spend thousands of dollars on marketing and advertising. The landscape and the laws of marketing treatment facilities and filling beds is changing. The thinking has changed, the terminology has changed, even the definition of addiction has changed. You work hard to get the proper clients into your programs.

It's amazing how little training many individuals working in Call Centers have had prior to actually working the phones in the Call Center. Professionals must be prepared before they can execute properly in any position, in any industry. When it comes to saving lives, and keeping a facility open by keeping the beds filled with the proper clients, you would think and hope that training would be paramount. The current landscape in the treatment industry demands that all professionals working in the industry know the importance of ethics in the workplace.

Best-Selling Author, Rev. Dr. Kevin T. Coughlin Ph.D. developed the curriculum for Call Center and Ethics training by sharing the strategies, skill sets, tools, and techniques that worked for him and his staff, and other interventionists, Directors, Owners, Therapists, Counselors, and CEOs for over two decades. Rev. Dr. Kevin T. Coughlin Ph.D. has created a program to help professionals to fill beds with the clients that need them, always keeping ethics as a priority with each and every client and their family.

Rev. Dr. Coughlin has already trained hundreds of addiction professionals on the fundamentals and techniques of Call Center and Ethics including counselors, therapists, recovery coaches, techs, CEOs, Owners, Interventionists, and entire teams at facilities. The results have always been the same; the owners, CEOs, and Directors have been amazed at what they didn't know about operating a successful, ethical call center.

This Amazing Book has already helped many individual professionals and facilities and ultimately has helped those who need treatment to find the correct facility, and to stay in treatment. Get your copy today and arm yourself with the knowledge and tools you will need to be successful!

Visit Rev. Dr. Coughlin's website at www.theaddiction.expert to sign up for his mailing list, information on new book releases, and live events.

Disclaimer: In this book, the author shares his experience, strength, and hope with readers, this should not be considered advice. All information in this book is for informational and educational purposes, not medical or psychiatric advice or to prescribe the use of any technique as a form of treatment for medical or psychiatric problems without the advice of a physician, psychiatrist or appropriate licensed professional either directly or indirectly. In the event, you use any of the information in this book for yourself, neither the authors nor the publisher accepts responsibility for your actions.

Call Center Agent Training

Call Center Professional Agent Training Platform will empower your customer service staff, call center agents, and all associates on the team with the skills they need to raise customer satisfaction levels, reduce conflict, and improve teamwork. This will lead to a more productive company and a healthy bottom line.

The Addiction and Recovery Field has never been more exciting than it is today. We are experiencing new modalities and changes in Treatment and aftercare. Call center agents have never been more important in helping to find placement for those that are sick and suffering find the correct facility where they can get the help that they so desperately need. More than one-hundred people a day are dying from overdoses in the United States.

New laws for addiction treatment marketing are on the horizon. Patient brokering is illegal and unethical, it will not be tolerated in any way, shape, or form. It is your responsibility to know the law, even if you are new to the industry. It is paramount for Owners, CEOs, Directors, and other personnel to understand the new landscape and to adopt ethical marketing and operating practices. The new era will bring much needed regulation and help everyone in the treatment industry to understand the new laws and any new licensing requirements for marketers. We will see true professionals in the treatment industry who are qualified to make assessments and put the client's needs first.

The days of paying to put heads in beds are over, it is unethical and illegal! Clients have the right to be placed in a facility that is best suited to care for their needs. For example, if John X. is an opiate addict and also suffers from an eating disorder; he should be placed in a facility that specializes in both opiate addiction and eating disorders. If Catherine B. is a pathological gambler and suffers from alcoholism, she should be placed in a facility that specializes in pathological gambling disorders and alcoholism. Clients should be able to utilize their insurance first to cover the cost of their treatment. Clients and their families should be dealt with honestly and not just told anything to close the deal for the facility of the Call Center Agent.

Privacy

Any medical information that an agent gathers from a client is personal and confidential. All facilities must be committed to protecting their client's medical information. Representatives of the company are not to give out any personal information to anyone except the client without prior written authorization. This includes immediate family members. The agent should be able to provide information on privacy release forms to clients to allow the release of information to specific individuals.

It is your responsibility to stay informed on your State's ethics codes, privacy laws, duty to report, Federal laws such as HIPAA laws. It's a good idea to consult with your attorney before going into business. You will also want to carry liability insurance. Use the professionals for their respective fields, for example, an Attorney for law issues, contracts, forming a corporation, an accountant for tax related issues, an insurance agent for liability insurance, etc. We are in a time of change, so most of these laws are changing. I will give you some websites on the resource page to assist you.

Agents must be oriented on the basics of the facility.

Agents should be introduced to the executive team, the management team, and all department heads.

They should have a clear understanding on policies including payroll, benefits, vacation policies, etc.

Agents also should understand scheduling, break policies, protocols for after work, work rules, etc.

Agents should have a clear understanding of safety and security policies.

Agents should have a clear understanding of dress code, parking rules, and where to find needed information when questions arise.

Agents should be educated on the company's mission, culture, vision, and core values. Agents are the voice and often the face of the company and must be trained well. They can't execute or help facilitate the process for overall company success if they don't know what the company is all about.

Agent training is paramount! If your company does a poor job on agent training, the customers will get subpar service at best. Your agents should be trained by experts; they must be prepared before they can execute in their positions. Encourage questions with agents and company leadership as well as their trainers.

Agents must be provided with comprehensive training on call center software. In order for the agents to be able to interact effectively with your clients, agents must be trained on how to effectively utilize your call center software. Your own in-house expert can do this training. Your company should have training manuals prepared for all new-hire agents to learn the basics. A trainer should walk agents through some of the more common scenarios that take place on a regular day; such as, joining conference calls, note editing, transferring calls outside of the department, adding management to a call, how to troubleshoot when common problems arise.

Agents should have a clear understanding of the company's client base, so they will be able to field questions and meet client needs adequately. Is there demographic information that can help the agent to do their job? A certain income level, age group, etc.

Call center agents should be educated on metrics that will be valued and tracked. This requires that the agents know what the metrics are and also how they are calculated, how they can access them and how they can improve them. All too often, management throws call-center agents on the phones before they are trained or ready. This is a costly mistake! It will most often lead to subpar service, frustrated and angry customers, and agent confusion. Providing in-depth training for call center agents will have a huge payout in the long run.

Agent Responsibility

Integrity	Legal Compliance
Competence	Mandatory Reporting
Ethics	Self-Disclosure
Standards	Non-Discrimination
Principles	Boundary Management
Quality	Harm Prevention
Respect	Conflicts of Interest
Professionalism	Confidentiality

Becoming an Excellent Call Center Agent

Take responsibility for your actions setting clear boundaries and follow the law!

1. Informed Consent: Roles, Rights, and Responsibilities, Duration of Relationship & Fees.

2. Competence and Established Theory: Practice only within Trained and Certified Scope.

3. Confidentiality: No unauthorized disclosure. (HIPAA)

4. Duty to Warn/Protect: People who are in imminent harm.

5. Minors and Families: All states require reporting of minors in danger of imminent harm.

6. Maintaining Appropriate Boundaries: Keep Professional Boundaries.

7. Counselor Self-Disclosure: Only reveal intimate self-information when appropriate.

8. Touch: Appropriate rule of thumb, don't.

9. Sexual Attraction: Don't get involved.

10. Recovery Boundaries: keep clear and professional boundaries.

11. Supervision: Everyone needs sounding boards a Mentor, a Coach.

12. Honoring Diverse Values: Respect the client's values within the framework of your job.

Only Licensed Clinicians diagnose! If you write a letter for a client about your Professional relationship, make sure you use the words, "in my opinion" or "it is my opinion" before making a statement.

HIPAA LAW: The Standards for Privacy of Individually Identifiable Health Information ("Privacy Rule") establishes, for the first time, a set of national standards for the protection of certain health information. The U.S. Department of Health and Human Services ("HHS") issued the Privacy Rule to implement the requirement of the Health Insurance Portability and Accountability Act of 1996 ("HIPAA"). 1 The Privacy Rule standards address the use and disclosure of individuals' health information—called "protected health information" by organizations subject to the Privacy Rule — called "covered entities," as well as standards for individuals' privacy rights to understand and control how their health information is used. Within HHS, the Office for Civil Rights ("OCR") has responsibility for implementing and enforcing the Privacy Rule with respect to voluntary compliance activities and civil money penalties.

New Laws and Landscape in Treatment

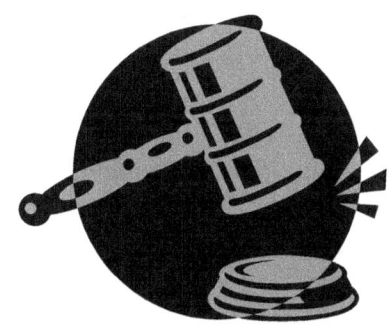

Patient Brokering Bills Now Law

HB 807 (SB 788) — Marketers will now have to be licensed and there are stiff penalties and fines for patient brokering, and centers will be help legally liable for deceptive marketing practices. It makes DCF the "big brother" and enforcer of the industry.

HB 249 (SB 588) — Paramedics, emergency techs, and hospitals to collect data on overdoses and report them to the Dept. of Health. Forces hospitals to adapt overdose protocols.

HB 477 — Directly attacks drug dealers with min. and mandatory jail time including heavy fines for dealing in fentanyl. It also gives prosecutors the option of imposing murder charges.

HB 557 (SB 840) — Directed toward prescribing physicians controlling the quantity of opioids prescribed to five days. The Prescriptions that are filled for any controlled substances must be reported in the State prescription drug monitoring database within one day.

SB 886 (HB 791) — Protects individuals that have been Marchman Acted by making their court records confidential.

Florida Lawmakers may set the tone for the Nation with these Bills that are now Florida Law.

Problem-Solving 101

Dealing with people on a regular basis, you will need a solid strategy for handling difficult situations. All it takes is good techniques to diffuse your client's anger. Remember, don't take things personally! Remember to smile. Be warm, friendly, and genuine. Don't feed into the client's drama!

Techniques to diffuse Angry Clients
1. Apologize and acknowledge that you hear the client and understand their feelings.
2. Sympathize, validate their feelings of frustration.
3. Accept Responsibility.
4. Prepare to help the client.

Example:
Mrs. Jones, I'm so sorry that we couldn't find a detox bed for John today.
I know that it must be very frustrating and disappointing for you both!
I promise you that I will personally work on John's case until it's resolved, again, my name is Amy and I'm here to help you.
I will get started right now looking for an open bed in all of the facilities that we use.

Tips
Don't tell clients what you can't do; tell them what you can do!
One-word answers are considered cold and uncaring.
Use proper English on the phone.
Be professional.
E-mail, telephone, and in person manners apply.
Say something fun, nice, and appropriate, get excited!
Frontline Fundamentals: Great customer service skills are critical to frontline training. Spoken communication skills (what you say and how you say it) make all the difference in the close.

Active Listening is the greatest Communication Tool Agents Have!

Listen to what the client says.

The greatest communication tool we have is active listening.
Pay attention to tones and inflections, they will tell you more than the words that the client speaks.
Be professional at all times.
Take notes on the conversation.
Always have extra pens or pencils and writing tablets.
Don't argue with clients.
Sometimes no matter how hard you try to help someone, they just won't appreciate your efforts. Don't take it personally, they're frustrated.
You won't be able to solve all problems, that's a fact of business.
Do the best you can!

Communication with Clients.

There is no doubt that the most problematic cause of misunderstandings is the lack of awareness of the concerns of others. If you want to avoid outcomes that are negative, you must follow certain guidelines or basic rules. The agent must be trained on the proper techniques and aware of the best methods to utilize the skill sets that they will learn during this training.

Ethics

A code of ethical conduct for Trained Professionals should be followed by all Professional Practitioners. The following rules of conduct demonstrates the minimum acceptable standards of conduct which all Professional Practitioners are expected to utilize as a clear guide to ethical behavior and responsibilities within their assigned duties. All Professionals are expected to follow local, state, and federal law.

Sections

FRC: Fraud Related Conduct 1.0	**SFY:** Safety & Welfare 6.0
PROS: Professional Standards 2.0	**CONF:** Confidentiality 7.0
SMIS: Sexual Misconduct 3.0	**UNL**: Unlawful Conduct 8.0
EXC: Exploitation of Clients 4.0	**RK**: Record Keeping 9.0
AUP: Assisting Unqualified Practice 5.0	**COI**: Cooperation with Investigation 10.0

Code of Ethical Conduct

Fraud Related Conduct

FRC 1.1: A Professional shall not be involved in any false or fraudulent claim, or provide any proof of such claim, to be paid under contract or insurance certificate benefit. Shall not present any false paperwork, or affidavit, or certificate. Seek to have another party commit or assist in an act of commission or omission to conduct fraud.

FRC1.2: A Professional shall not use misrepresentation in the procurement of certification, falsification of references, work history, experience, or professional qualifications.

FRC1.3: A Professional shall not use a title, credential, license, firm name, letterhead, publication, document which implies an ability, relationship, or qualification that they are not entitled to use.

FRC1.4: A Professional shall not knowingly sign a false document, and shall not provide service under a false name.

FRC1.5: A Professional must not create and publish false advertisement.

FRC1.6: A Professional who participates in the writing, editing, or publishing of professional papers, media resources, brochures, or books must preserve the integrity of the profession by acknowledging and documenting used in production.

Professional Standards

PROS2.1: A Professional shall not participate in discrimination of any type for any reason.

PROS2.2: A Professional shall comply with all terms, conditions, expectations, and limitations of any certification or license the Professional may hold.

PROS2.3: A Professional shall not engage in any conduct that does not meet accepted standards of competence required by law.

PROS2.4: A Professional shall not perform services outside of the scope of their credentials, training, expertise, and competence. The Professional Practitioner shall refer to a qualified Professional.

PROS2.5: A Professional shall honor and protect confidence following state and federal law as required.

PROS2.6: The Professional shall get the appropriate releases signed as deemed necessary prior to any discloser except as authorized or required by law.

PROS2.7: The Professional Practitioner shall not discontinue service to a client without proper closer and or referral.

PROS2.8: The Professional shall obtain an appropriate consultation or make a proper referral when the client's problem is beyond the Professional's scope of expertise.

Sexual Misconduct

SMIS 3.1: A Professional shall not engage in romantic/sexual activities or romantic/sexual contact with clients, whether such contact is consensual or not. This applies to in person and electronic interactions/relationships.

SMI 3.2: A Professional shall not provide services to individuals with whom they have had a prior sexual relationship. This applies to in person and electronic interactions/relationships.

SMI3.3: A Professional shall not engage in sexual activities or sexual contact with former clients when there is a risk of exploitation or potential harm to the client. This applies to in person and electronic interaction/relationships.

SMI3.4: A Professional shall not knowingly engage in romantic/sexual activities or romantic/sexual contact with clients' relatives or other individuals with whom clients maintain a close personal relationship when there is a risk of exploitation or potential harm to the client. This applies to in person and electronic interactions/relationships.

Exploitation of Clients

EXC 4.1: A Professional shall not misappropriate property from clients and/or family members of clients.

EXC 4.2: A Professional shall neither ask for nor accept favors, free services, gifts of substantial monetary value or gifts that impair the integrity or efficacy of the service relationship.

EXC 4.3: A Professional shall not develop, implement, condone or maintain exploitative relationships with clients and/or family members of clients. This applies in person and to electronic interactions/relationships.

EXC4.4: A Professional shall not offer, give, or receive commissions, rebates, or any other forms of remuneration for a client referral.

EXC4.5: A Professional shall not accept fees or gratuities for professional work from a person who is entitled to such services through an institution and/or agency by which the Professional Practitioner is employed.

Assisting Unqualified / Unlicensed Practice

AUP 5.1: A Professional shall not refer a client to a person that he/she knows or should have known is not qualified by training, experience, certification, or license to perform the delegated professional responsibility.

Safety & Welfare

SFY 6.1: A Professional shall not consume any psychoactive substance to the extent or in such manner as to be dangerous or injurious to the professional, a recipient of services, to any other person, or to the extent that such use of any psychoactive substance impairs the ability of the professional to safely perform their duties.

SFY 6.2: Where a Professional is determined to be a mandated reporter (i.e., abuse and/or neglect) by country law they are required to comply with all mandatory reporting requirements and have an obligation to be aware of these requirements.

SFY 6.3: When a client is in clear and imminent danger to self-harm with serious bodily injury or death, a Professional shall consistent with state and federal confidentiality laws, take reasonable steps to protect the client.

SFY 6.4: *All certified Professionals are mandated child abuse reporters!

Confidentiality

CONF7.1: Professionals shall make every effort to protect the confidentiality of their clients and follow all State, and Federal laws including but not limited to HIPAA.

Unlawful Conduct

UNL8.1: Once certified, a Professional shall not be convicted of any crime relating to the individual's ability to provide services as determined by local state licensing Boards.
UNL8.2: A Professional shall not be convicted of any crime that involves the sale or trafficking of any controlled or psychoactive substance, driving while impaired, driving under the influence, theft, sexual misconduct, or fraud. This includes internet crimes.

Record Keeping

RK 9.1: A Professional shall keep timely and accurate records consistent with current standards of best practices and shall not falsify, amend, or knowingly make incorrect entries or fail to make timely essential entries into the client record.

Cooperation with Investigation / Reporting Violations

COI 10.1: A Professional should cooperate in any investigation conducted pursuant to this Code of Ethical Conduct. Professionals shall not interfere with any investigation or proceedings, shall not misrepresent facts or make false statements, destroy evidence, or harass or threaten witnesses.
COI 10.2: A Professional shall report violations of professional conduct of other certified professionals to the appropriate licensing/disciplinary authority when he/she knows or should have known that another Professional Practitioner has violated ethical standards and has failed to take corrective action after an informal intervention.
COI 10.1: Any Professional who is under investigation or involved in a disciplinary proceeding, or has been sanctioned, arrested/convicted of a crime in another jurisdiction must notify their local state, and/or federal licensing Board immediately.

The exact Ethical Standards varies State to State and Company to Company; the above listed standards are to be used only as an example of minimum standards and guidelines. Make sure to check with any licensing Boards and State Boards for the Ethical Standards that you will be expected to follow based on your credentials, position, and company.

Professional Practitioners don't do any process work, that's what therapists and counselors do. Example: A therapist says, "Alice how did that make you feel at the time?" The counselor says, "When you were abused back in 1990, how did you feel?" Our Professionals work in the day moving forward. Example: The Practitioner says, "Mary, what are you going to do today about your problem?" "John, let's make an action plan for the next month to combat your addiction." See the difference? Only work within the boundary of what you are trained and licensed to do in your position. Never work outside of the scope of your training and licensing.

A basic set of core ethical guidelines for professionals cannot be taken lightly, although many guidelines are yet to be established for the new and growing field of professional practitioners. The ability to recognize and respond to ethical dilemmas, while clients and their families have so many needs, is a complex task even for seasoned veterans and experienced masters.

Call Center Training with Scripts

Today's behavioral health marketplace is highly competitive. Strong relationships with strategic partners and key referral resources have never been more important. A company's reputation and integrity is absolutely critical.

Marketing and business development staff drive business, while the call center staff must close the deal! Most often, the call center staff will create the first impression of the business for the client. This entire experience is magnified and reviewed and has the potential to generate a great deal of additional word-of-mouth referrals. Call center representatives who field intake calls must have in-depth knowledge of the facility, addiction and recovery modalities and principles, insurance plans, detoxification, process addictions, co-occurring disorders, the judicial system including parole and probation, a problem-solving nature, great interpersonal and communication skills including active listening and powerful questioning, understand family dynamics, and the addicted mind.

Call Center Scripts for Employees:

Scripts for Call Centers.

Call center scripts represent what should be said while communicating with a new referral or customer. Call center agents who would otherwise struggle with the delivery of key ideas, learn everything from greetings to customer service, delivering a polished and professional script to help them to seal deals that they might otherwise lose.

Well-written scripts can help agents to be more fluid and professional during their conversations with potential clients. Poorly designed scripts will have negative effects on closings.

The perfect script can guarantee a smooth call and will provide the agent with all of the crucial information needed to hook the client and close the deal. Some agents need more help than others when it comes to expressing their thoughts and organizing their words. Scripting will ensure that the agent can express their thoughts and words in the most eloquent manner, expressing confidence to the client.

For most clients, the call center agent is the primary point of contact with your Treatment center. The interactions among call center agent and clients can have a significant impact on people's perception of your company, positive or negative. The agent can have a tremendous impact on your bottom line! Doesn't it seem clear that it is a very smart investment to train the call center agents? Yes, it certainly does!

For any business, good customer service makes all the difference in the world. Good communication leads to consistency and teamwork. All these factors lead to a successful business.

Here are some examples of Bad Scripts:

1. Repetition.
2. A script is too mechanical, too verbose.
3. Measuring call in time instead of key performance metrics.
4. Admitting self-fault immediately, or criticizing or blaming the client.
5. Overly friendly introductions and/or over polite scripts.

When it comes to Call Centers for Treatment we are dealing with Life and Death! People's well-being comes first; the money will follow. We have the responsibility to get the client safe and into the appropriate facility with the appropriate level of care.

To maximize the efficiency of your call center, scripts must be designed to efficiently and effectively handle the needs of the incoming caller. A successful call center is one where an agent fulfills a customer's need and at the same time generates or retains revenue from the customer.

Tips for building effective call center scripts:

1. The goal of every script is to close the client.
2. Research about your clients, their needs and how you can most help them before developing your script.
3. Develop goals and continually track the performance of your scripts. How many of your leads do you close each week and each month?

While developing a call center script, make sure to keep it simple to operate and edit while necessary.

A successful sales call is a call that is well planned and organized.

You don't want your script content to get outdated! Script content must be carefully revised and updated constantly.

Tones and inflections are very important to your communication with clients. Make sure your script has the appropriate tone for the situation and does not sound like reading a textbook. It should be accurate, clear, and interesting.

A perfect script is one that allows for an appropriate response to any given client interaction and prompts the call agent to stay consistent with the company message.

Practice writing a script for a treatment center:
Good afternoon:

Try writing another script in the space below:

How do you think your script sounds?

Does it sound natural?

Did you say what you wanted to say?

Do you think it will help close the deal?

Remember to be honest and ethical, putting the client's needs first, this is a must. When you are honest and caring with clients, they will pick up on those facts and it will help you to do your job. If you were the client would you want to hear from a pushy car salesman type of agent or an honest and caring agent who is knowledgeable and only wants what is best for you or your family member in need? The answer here is clear!

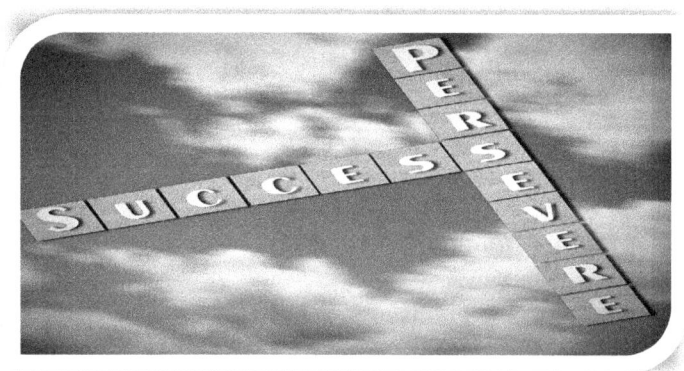

80/20 Rule

80% of calls answered within 20 seconds.
More Agents
More Cost
Competitive Market
Higher Service Level
Cost Customer Appreciates Service Levels
Rise and Fall Together

Referral:

Establish and maintain relations with other professionals, agencies, and community resources.
Continuously assess and evaluate.
Clarifying expectations and client follow-through.
Exchange information with the referral agency or professional.
Respect confidentiality, ethics, and responsibility.
Evaluate the outcome of the referral.

Engagement:

Case finding and pretreatment
Reaching out to the client
Identify immediate needs (triage)
Motivation while awaiting treatment
Certain cases have simultaneous life needs (such as inmates)
Meet criminal justice requirements
Anger management

Clarify Expectations of Treatment:

Reduce roadblocks to treatment:

(1) Motivational interviewing
(2) Addiction and recovery education
(3) Consequences of substance abuse
(4) Basic survival needs
(5) Case manager-client relationship based on trust
(6) Prescreening for program eligibility

Assessment should include serious problematic behaviors, indications of self-harm or harm to others:

Self-mutilation (cutter)
Suicide attempts
Criminal record (supervision of CJS)
Violent behaviors
Eating disorders
Sex Addicts: Do they have to report if convicted of a sex crime (Will face discrimination.)

Service Coordination:
Implement the treatment plan.
Initiate collaboration with referral source.
Review screening, assessment information.
Confirm the client's eligibility for admission.
Admission to treatment.

Making Sure Clients Get the Correct level of Care

Communicate information with the client (and family with signed release documentation) the following:

Treatment nature of services.
Program goals and objectives, and procedures.
Rules for client conduct.
Treatment daily schedule.
Costs of treatment, payment schedule, and acceptable forms of payment.
Client's rights and responsibilities.
Coordinate all treatment services provided to the client by all resources.

Primary treatment:

Examine the damage of addiction in all areas of the addict's life.
A bio-psychosocial assessment is necessary.
Pairing clients with the appropriate treatment modalities.
Five categories of primary treatment:
Early intervention
Outpatient services
Intensive outpatient or partial hospitalization
Residential or inpatient service
Medically managed intensive inpatient services

Referral, Engagement, and Assessment:

1. You receive a referral for a client who needs Treatment.

2. The caller is a relative of the addicted person (Could also be a spouse or parent), a referral resource, or the client.

3. What do you ask the relative, referral resource, or client during the initial conversation?

Ask for the caller's full name and a call back number? In case the call drops, you will be able to call the client back.

Ask the name of the addicted person? Call them by name during the conversation. Example: "Based on what you're telling me it seems clear that Sue will need detox."

What is the addicted person's drug of choice? When did they last use? How much did they use? How often do they Use? Do they use any other illicit drugs or alcohol? When did they first start using? This information will help you to start to form a picture as to needs for treatment.

Does the addicted person have a mental health diagnosis? If yes, what is it? Are they prescribed any medication for the problem or for any other reason? If yes, what medications are they taking? This will further help you to assess needs for placement. Some facilities don't allow certain medications.

Is the addicted person a cutter, have they attempted suicide in the past, do they have an eating disorder? Important information for placement and safety.

Does the addicted person have any legal trouble? If yes, what is it? Have they ever been arrested? Are they on parole or probation? If yes, in what state? What is the officer's name? What were they arrested for, the original charges? Do they have any active warrants? Do they have any history of violence? This information is very important! If they have an active warrant and you place them, you could get into trouble for aiding a wanted person! If on parole or probation they will need permission to leave the state or go into certain counties within their own state, or they may be violated and arrested. You will want to know the original charges because if they are convicted of arson, rape, murder, serious assaults, sex crimes certain facilities and communities will not take them. They may also need specialized treatment.

What is the addicted person's age and gender? For placement, you need to know this information. If a minor, you need permission to take the addicted person over state lines. (More liability comes with under age clients.)

What kind of physical health is the addicted person in? Are they ambulatory? You need to know if there are any special circumstances for placement. If the person is handicapped if they have HIV/Aids, or any other special needs.

Has the addicted person ever gone into treatment before? If yes, what type, detox, residential, outpatient, counseling, etc.? What was the result and why? Helps you to know who you're dealing with.

Has the addicted person ever had detox complications in the past? If yes, what were they? Important to know for safety issues.

Is the addicted person covered by any form of insurance? You will need to know this for placement.

Does the addicted person live with the caller? If not, where do they live? Get both addresses. You will need this information moving forward.

Is the addicted person willing to get help? This will help you determine if an intervention is needed.

Does the addicted person have a job, housing, or any special needs? Information you need to do your job. (Example: pregnant females, HIV positive clients have special needs. Some facilities won't take certain special needs clients.)

Who or what is the funding resource for the addicted person? You need to know this to see what they can afford.

Where is the addicted person now? Are they willing to talk to you? Gives you vital information. (Always follow up immediately, or risk losing clients.)

If you are able to talk with the addicted person, you should be able to get more information. Perhaps more honest information as to drug use, maybe not. You can also find out more about family dynamics. The more information you get, the more it will help you to make informed decisions as to placement.

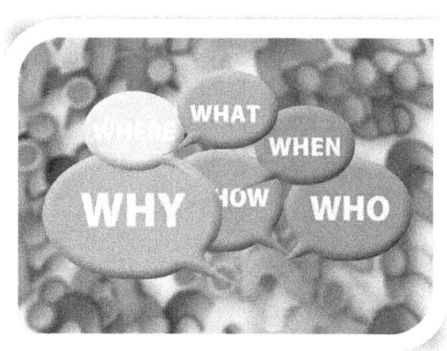

Addiction and Treatment

MODELS OF ADDICTION:

Minnesota Model: Twelve-Step, Disease Model, World View is Changing.
Florida Model: ½ way and ¾ Housing, Aftercare PHP, IOP Therapy, REF, AA & NA based Disease Model, Urine Testing.
Smart Recovery: Self-Empowerment, Harm Reduction, Coping Skills, Compulsions.
Christian Tract: Spiritual, Faith Based, Prayer, Meditation, twelve-Step.
Holistic: Fitness, Yoga, Meditation.
Scientology: All Empowering Methodologies.

STYLES OF TREATMENT:

Detox: Removal of Drugs from the system, or placed on medication management $20,000+ Ins.
Inpatient: Goal to remain sober, Twenty-Eight Days $12,000-$63,000 Ins. and OOP
PHP: Partial Hospitalization Program: Day Treatment, Usually Thirty Days, $10,000-$30,000 INS and OOP.
IOP: Intensive Outpatient Program: six-week evening program, three times a week for three hours, $8,000-$30,000 Ins. and OOP.
Halfway House: Usually six months: curfew, zero tolerance, drug testing, $150-$500 weekly OOP only.
Meetings AA/NA: Sponsorship, Home Group, Zero Tolerance Free.
Recovery Coach: Hourly, Daily, Weekly, stays with client, can go with client to events or where needed. $125 Hourly $600-$1,500 Daily OOP Only.
Sober Companion: Similar to Recovery Coach, usually hired for specific event or min. of thirty days, $350-$1,500 a day, OOP only.
Case Manager: Manages from Referral to Disengagement, $250-$2,000 a Day.

MODELS OF TREATMENT:

Abstinence: Zero Tolerance.
Twelve-Step AA/NA Abstinence with Meetings, Steps.
Faith Oriented: Specific Religious, Zero Tolerance.
Moderation Management: some but not primary Drug of choice.
Holistic: Fitness, wellness, health, Alternative Therapies.
Medication Management: Suboxone, Methadone, Vivitrol, etc.

Types of special needs clients:

Homelessness
Acute physical problems/ Handicapped
HIV/ AIDS
Mental Illness
Poverty
Inmates/ Sex Offenders
Sexual Orientation
Elderly
Adolescence/ Parents of young children

Admissions Procedure Manual:

Phase I:

Initial point of contact
Call
Click
E-mail
Gather brief clinical and all insurance info
Doc, MH, prior TX history etc.
Client Name
Client DOB
Primary Insured Name
Primary Insured DOB
Insurance Type
Id #
Group #
800 # for Behavioral Health Services
Address
Employer

Phase II:

Client doesn't have OON benefit or no insurance? No problem…
What type of insurance? For example: PPO, POS, HMO, EPO, Medicare, Medicaid
Gather same info listed in section 2 of Phase I
No get into ACTION!

For Insurance clients:

Call insurance company and get verification of benefits (VOB)
Will the client meet medical necessity? If so for what level…Detox, Residential, PHP, IOP, OP
Client's VOB results include co-pay, deductible, coinsurance, OOP max, exclusions etc.
Submit VOB and Clinical to Admissions Director for approval of admission

Phase III:

Customer Acquisition and Conversion Optimization
Contact client, client's family, or referring professional with final decision
Arrange the logistics of a bed to bed transfer
Where is client...home, hospital/detox, crisis center, treatment center
Will the client need transportation?
When will the client be ready to admit?
How will the client be funding treatment...Insurance, PP, Other?
Confirm with family, or referral partner upon client's arrival.

Follow-up

When to follow-up? Immediately, and continually until admission.

How to follow-up? Polite, enthusiastic and willing to go to any lengths to help 24/7 365.

Why follow-up? The client's life is on the line and remember they may not admit immediately continue to follow-up.

What is the next step? Take care of your client's families and referral sources and always strive to work in conjunction to the outside business development reps (they work extremely hard to produce these vital leads in this competitive market space), clinical team, and everyone else involved.

Admissions Procedure Manual Key:

DOC: drug of choice
MH: mental health
TX: treatment
DOB: date of birth
BEH: behavioral
OON: out of network benefit –good insurance for example: PPO, POS
PPO: Preferred provider organization –can go anywhere TX (30+ days)
POS: Point of service –can go anywhere for TX (30+ days)
HMO: Health Maintenance Organization. –has to stay in-network (shorter stays usually between 7-14 days)
EPO: Exclusive provider organization –similar to HMO in-network benefit only (short stays between 7-14 days.)
VOB: Verification of benefits
RES: residential TX

PHP: partial hospitalization program (Florida model provides community housing component)
IOP: intensive outpatient program (Florida model provides community housing component)
OP: outpatient program (Florida model provides community housing component)
OOP max: out of pocket max that member is responsible after co-pay and deductible is met)
Exclusions: the results of the VOB will reveal if there are any exclusions in insurance benefit, for example, certain policies will not have a RES benefit or PHP or IOP etc.

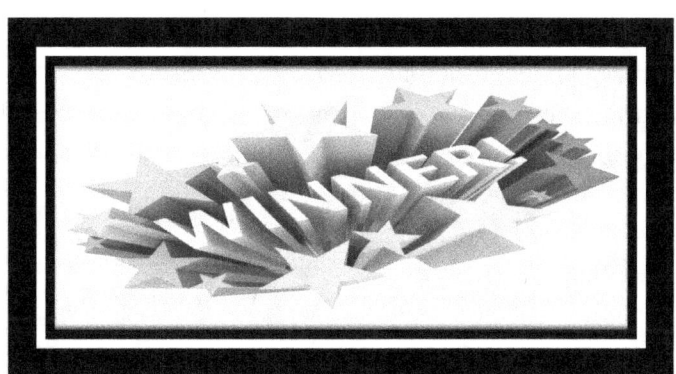

The Art of Closing a Deal

Everything is important from the first impression you make or engagement through to the signed contract! The agents who are successful consistently utilize a variety of skills, tools, and techniques that are tried, tested, and proven to work in the industry.

1. You must know your product, services, and/or facility and every aspect about them.

Be prepared to answer any question a potential client may ask. Practice in the mirror, with coworkers, friends, and family. First impressions are critical to the outcome!

Be confident and utilize your time with the potential client to the fullest.
Remember to smile when meeting face-to-face, give a firm handshake and look the potential client in the eye.
Body language, tones, and inflections are very important.
Avoid too much small talk; you control the conversation.

2. Make sure to speak loud and clear. Be prepared.

Guide the client through any presentations you may be utilizing. Keep good posture.
Come to a logical conclusion that the client can't help but agree with.

3. Show the client that you're an expert in the field: relay information by memorizing statistics.

For example, over a hundred Americans die each day from opiate abuse. Fatal overdoses in the past fifteen years have more than doubled. Since 1999, fatal overdoses from opiate medications have quadrupled. Twenty-three million people need treatment for addiction, only three million seek it.

You need to blend the statistics with charm.
You will want to humanize your presentation by asking rhetorical questions and using relative statements.

4. You need to control the mood of the call, room, meeting, etc.

Think about what emotion you want to convey. Don't ever be confrontational. You need to be a master at reading body language, not just using your own.

The potential client must see you as their friend, not their enemy.

5. Make sure that you're organized in every way.

If for some reason the potential client comes up with a question that you really don't know, don't fake it!
Tell them that you are not sure, but you will find out ASAP and get them the correct answer.

6. If you are professional and respectful, the potential client will be convinced by you that they are in good hands and the close will be yours.

They will want to help you. They will feel like you're all one team.

Always be on time.
Be professional and respectful.

7. Make the deal happen if you can.

If a potential client's mother says, "I'll bring my son in Monday after the Holiday; I don't have time before then." Tell her that the facility will send a driver to pick her son up this afternoon. Make the close happen. Time is not your friend; too much could happen over the weekend to lose the close. More importantly, the son could die!

Whatever the person's reason is not to close; look for an immediate solution without being pushy or rude.
You might talk about how short the window of opportunity is with those addicted to drugs to be willing to get help after hitting a bottom. Then when they get comfortable in their own skin again, that window slams shut! The best case is to bring them in right away if they are willing. Talk about how awful it would be if they went on one last binge on the weekend and overdosed! It will make perfect sense to the mother and she will close.

8. Practice Makes Perfect!

Role-play and practice scripts and talking as often as you can until you feel you can do it backward and in your sleep. The confidence will show and the customers will like it.

Just utilizing these few tips will make a large impact on your ability to close deals.

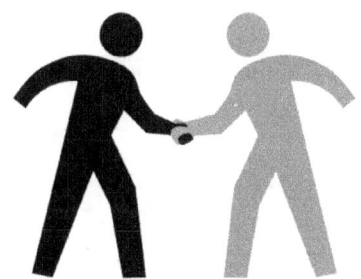

The Psychological Reasons People Make Decisions

To convert leads into customers it's important that you understand the psychological reasons people make decisions and choices when and why they do.

Pleasure and Pain.

Human behavior is driven by the desire for pleasure and the need to avoid all forms of pain.
When human beings do something that seems painful it is because they associate pleasure with such an action.
You must be able to understand your potential customer; who are they, what influences them?
What influences do they already have in their lives?
Once you identify who your niche customer is and what is their goal?
Then you can move potential clients close to their goal in your message before attempting to close.
When you are close to their goal they are very likely to close to achieve their goal.
A completed goal equals pleasure; your company equals pleasure.

Give Clients Explanations.

People want answers.
People seek to understand everything.
If you explain why you are offering something from your company, you are more likely to have success in closing.

Be Creative.

Pleasure potential makes people want it.
People want new, fresh ideas, products.

Keep It Simple.

People always will gravitate to the simplest solution to achieve a result.
Show your client's your simple program or blueprint to get to solution.
The problem always defines the solution.
There is always a solution; however, there are perception and perspective problems that block solutions.

Share an experience.

Sharing stories with others affect the senses and emotions.
This will fire the client's emotional brain. (Same area of the brain that closes.)
Helps people feel like they have experiences that they haven't had.

Pick a common enemy and use it.

In addiction, you have a built-in enemy, the disease of addiction itself.
You and the client become teammates against the common enemy.
They will need you to defeat this powerful enemy.

Provide information that helps answer the client's questions about their goal.

Establish yourself as an expert in your business field.
Be prepared to answer all of the client's questions about their need and your company.
When you answer what they want to know, they will feel pleasure.
Inspire the client's curiosity in some way will help to close.

Make your potential client's feel important.

We all need to feel important to our peers in some way.
Show your clients that you care.
A key here is excellent customer service, showing value and making them more likely to close.

Community is important to all people.

We all have a need to feel connected to others.
It makes us feel secure and comfortable to be a part of a social community.
Help clients feel as though they will be a part of a community when they close.
When you build a community, they will drive your business for you.
Give client's something that makes them feel part of the community.

Use testimonies of other clients.

We are social beings.
Show your potential clients how others have benefited from using your services.
You can show potential clients the results through like-minded people's testimonials.
Have reference from former clients available both video and written.

Closing Deals

Have you identified the decision maker in the family?

If you're not talking directly to the decision maker, do whatever it takes to get them on the phone with you, or set up a meeting with them as soon as possible. This will lead to a much faster close.

Honesty, Genuine, and Real in your conversations.

If you sound rehearsed, fake, like a used-car salesman you will never close! Be honest and sincere, genuine, and real, people know when you are, they can sense these qualities in conversations. Let your client know that you care about them and their company's success. Never be cold and uncaring.

Know why clients don't close.

When you present to clients build in excuse busters that shoot down all of the reasons that clients don't buy. Take away their excuses before they say them. You need to brainstorm about this and plan your presentation carefully.

Explain to the client why it's important for them to make their decision now.

Addiction has a built-in sense of urgency.
Their loved one faces death, prison, and harm if they don't get help.
They need to go door to door from wherever they are because of the dangers.
Time is of the essence their loved one's life is at stake.

You're always a Professional!

Show the clients that you know your stuff, that you are an expert.
Keep things focused on your areas of knowledge.
Give them proof that you are an expert.

What is so special about you and your company?

Know how your company is different and better than others.
How are you and your company special?
What extra services do you provide to clients?
What makes you stand out from the crowd?
These are your real selling points and your clients want to know.
What is the main difference between you and your company and others?
What is your success rate?

Clients are more demanding and aware of the competitive market than ever before in history.

Don't look at yourself as a salesperson; you're a problem solver!
Clients want help to solve their problem and reach their goal.
If you can show the client a clear road map that you can help them get from point A to Z in a simple manner and at a reasonable price point, you should be able to close.

How do you get referrals?

Utilize your strongest relationships and ask for referrals.
Network with other professionals.
Utilize social media.
Former clients and word of mouth are your best resources.
Set up free informational webinars to show that you're the go to expert in the field.
Set up a website that gives people a reason to keep coming back on a regular basis that also shows that you are the expert that you are. Make it fresh and exciting!
Do live events where your niche clients are sure to be.
Do e-mail blasts through companies like "Constant Contact."
Do "giveaways" on your website in exchange for email addresses.

When you call is important.

Make your calls and call backs when you are likely to get the decision makers on the phone.
The best time to call statistically is 4:00 PM to 5:00 PM; second best 8:00 AM to 9:00 AM.
The worst time to call is 11:00 AM to 2:00 PM statistically.
Thursdays are the best day; Wednesdays second best statistically.
Tuesdays are the worst day statistically.
Thursdays between 4:00 PM and 5:00 PM you should be on fire!

Utilize social media to research clients.

When you have a new potential client Google them.
Check out their LinkedIn profile and Facebook.
Check out their website.
Find out what makes them tick; what are their priorities?
What will their excuses not to close be?
These facts will help you close.

How do you open a conversation?

Please don't use old, boring openings!
Try something new, fresh, exciting, humorous but professional.
"Can I have 3.5 minutes of your time?"
"Can we talk about your goals?"
Getting rid of old and boring increases your chances by up to 20%.

Build a relationship with the client.

Remember that active listening is the most powerful communication tool that human beings have.
Listen to the client don't cut them off. If they're talking, they won't hang up.
Make sure you introduce yourself and your company if you're talking to the client for the first time.

80% of clients don't close until approximately the 5th conversation with a professional.

Don't give up. Hang in there.
Between 45% and 50% (Approximately) of sales people quit trying after the first call, of one follow up call.
Don't leave the follow-up to the client, get their e-mail and their cell number so that you can follow-up with them.

When clients call.

Make sure that you answer, not a machine.
Greet your potential client with energy and a positive attitude.
Utilize powerful open-ended questions.
Use powerful words in your questions like why, what, how, when, who, where.
Paraphrase to show the client that you understand what they're saying to you.

Write down the results of your efforts.

Keep a log of calls and results; client name, what was discussed, contact info, follow-up info, etc., end results.
Keep track of your overall statistics so you know if your efforts are working or if you need to adjust something.

Never take things personally.

Sometimes people will be ruthless with you.
Don't take it personally; let it go when you hang up the phone.
Remember this is a numbers game, you can't win them all.
Don't let fear take over!

Voice.

Pay attention to your tones and inflections.
Say your words clearly and slowly so that the client can understand.
Don't rapid fire like a used-car salesman.
If in person, make sure that you smile and show warmth.
When using a script, keep it simple and direct, don't sound rehearsed.
Heave confidence, be polite, and be credible.

Be on the lookout for Blockers or gatekeepers.

When you call these are the people who answer and screen you from the real decision makers.
Leave a message for the decision maker to call you back.
Find out when the decision maker will be there so that you can call back.
Often decision makers are in late in the afternoon.

What does a client's caller ID read when you call?

Make sure that you are set to private.
You are at a disadvantage otherwise.
The curiosity alone will make the client answer.

Longer calls convert better than short calls do.

This generally means the client is comfortable with the call center agent.
Extroverts, enthusiastic, and ambitious helps make successful agents.
Confidence and building rapport with clients help agents convert.
Strong communication skills are a must for agents.

Owners, CEOs, and Managers should create healthy agent environments.

Motivating agents creates an environment of productivity.
Healthy competitions increase motivation.
Encourage agents to share successful tactics with each other.
Employee of the month builds individual and company pride within organizations.

What else do clients hear in the background?

Make sure that you call in a quiet area without background noise.
Clients should not be able to hear other agent's conversations.
There should be no distractions such as music or televisions playing.
There should not be conversations going on in the background where the agent is calling from.
Make sure that the client can hear the agent, speak up!

Call Center Agents should be cross-trained to answer difficult questions.

We live in a society where people want instant gratification.
If you can't answer their questions immediately, they will go find someone else who can.
Never guess at a question you don't know the answer to.
Be honest, tell them you don't know but you will get the answer for them and get right back to them A.S.A.P., never lie to a client!
There should be enough staff to handle peak times, 80-20 Rule.
Companies should utilize role-play to practice handling tough questions.
Prioritize urgent calls.

Agents should have an understanding of clients.

What is it like to stand in the client's shoes?
Agents must have an understanding of the problem of addiction, the solution, modalities of treatment, mental health, family support systems such as Al-Anon and Families Anonymous, Addiction support groups such as AA, and NA. aftercare, etc.

What skills do call center agents need to have?

The ability to think quickly.

Great communication skills: active listening and powerful questioning, understanding of body language 55% human communication, tones, and inflections 38% human communication, spoken word 7% human communication.

Persuasion skills.
Patience.
Knowledge of their business.
Computer skills.
Outgoing personalities.
Confidence.
Pleasant and clear voice.
Ability to steer conversations.
Writing skills.
Empathy.
Be strategic. Personable, and efficient.

Call centers are fast-paced.

The main factors are how quickly the agent answers the phone.
Customer service.
Resolving client goal coming to solution or closing.
At times, the agent will be under a tremendous amount of pressure.

Pay attention to detail and accuracy.

The clients are the backbone of your company.
Clients must trust that their call is being handled professionally and correctly.
Clients put their faith in the agent as the go-to expert to help solve their problem or goal.
Agents must be accurate, honest, and consistent.
Agents must continue to learn on a regular basis and retain the information.

Agents must learn to deal with difficult clients and problem solve.

Often clients will call because they are upset about something and want it fixed immediately.
It's the agent's job to diffuse the client quickly.
Learning skills to deal with complaints and difficult people is part of an agent's job.
Listening and paraphrasing will help a great deal.

Agents must learn to be flexible.

The phones must be answered.
You may be called in with short notice.
You may have to work Holidays and weekends.
Anything can happen, agents must be ready for any call.

Call-Center Agents need to be organized.

Agents must be able to multitask.
Agents must meet deadlines.
Agents must follow up on leads.
Follow up on initial calls that have not closed.
Organization can make all the difference to converting and the bottom line.

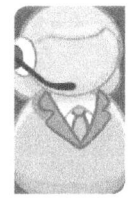

Twelve Closing Phrases that Make Deals Happen

"Is there any reason, if we offer you our services at this price today, that you wouldn't take advantage of our offer?"

"If we can find a way to deal with (Objection), would you commit to signing the contract today for a period of (set period of time)?"

"Would you like my help today?"

"So, when can we get started?"

"If we were to give you a (___%) discount would you sign the contract today?"

"Taking everything that we've discussed into consideration, I think these two options are the best for you. Would you like to go with thirty or ninety days?"

"I would hate to see your family have any more negative consequences because (_____) hasn't made the commitment to get the help that they need. Are you ready to take this crucial step to protect your family today?"

"Will you commit to this life changing decision today?"

"Our program is tried, tested, and proven, will you join us today?"

"Your new life can start today; are you ready for change?"

"We come well recommended; why don't you give us a try?"

"Let us help you today; make today the first day of a new and wonderful life!"

It's All About the Clients!

Remember that sales in the treatment industry do not equal shady, dishonest, or misleading! You must be ethical in all dealings with clients and other professionals in the industry.

Remember the client's needs come first if your facility is not the best fit for the client, refer them to a facility that is the best fit. For example: the client has an eating disorder and is a pathological gambler and your facility doesn't specialize in either of these problems, you would need to refer the client to a facility that does specialize in both these problems. Don't worry about the fact that you're giving away a client. You will be raising the bar ethically and the standards in your facility. Word will quickly get around that you care about clients and that they always come first; you will have more referrals than you know what to do with! Remember that the landscape of treatment has changed, the more honest, caring, and ethical facilities who put the client's lives first will be the most successful facilities. You want your facility to have an excellent name in the treatment industry. You want other professionals in the industry to feel 100% comfortable to refer clients to your facility. Give them good solid reasons to do so!

If someone is suicidal this is the number for the NSPL

**Call the National Suicide Prevention Lifeline

1-800-273-8255

Definitions

A call centre or call center: is a centralized office used for receiving or transmitting a large volume of requests by telephone. An inbound call centre is operated by a company to administer incoming product support or information inquiries from consumers. Outbound call centers are operated for telemarketing, solicitation of charitable or political donations, debt collection and market research. A contact centre is a location for centralized handling of individual communications, including letters, faxes, live support software, social media, instant message, and e-mail. A call centre has an open workspace for call centre agents, with workstations that include a computer for each agent, a telephone set/headset connected to a telecom switch, and one or more supervisor stations. It can be independently operated or networked with additional centers, often linked to a corporate computer network, including mainframes, microcomputers, and LANs. Increasingly, the voice and data pathways into the centre are linked through a set of new technologies called computer telephony integration. The contact centre is a central point from which all customer contacts are managed. Through contact centers, valuable information about the company are routed to appropriate people, contacts to be tracked and data to be gathered. It is generally a part of company's customer relationship management. A contact centre can be defined as a coordinated system of people, processes, technologies, and strategies that provides access to information, resources, and expertise, through appropriate channels of communication, enabling interactions that create value for the customer and organization. Contact centers, along with call centers and communication centers all fall under a larger umbrella labeled as the contact centre management industry. This is becoming a rapidly growing recruitment sector, as the capabilities of contact centers expand and thus require ever more complex systems and highly skilled operational and management staff. Most large companies use contact centers as a means of managing their customer interaction. These centers can be operated by either an in-house department responsible or outsourcing customer interaction to a third-party agency (known as Outsourcing Call Centers).

The Stark law: is a limitation on certain physician referrals. It prohibits physician referrals of designated health services ("DHS") for Medicare and Medicaid patients if the physician (or an immediate family member) has a financial relationship with that entity. 42 U.S.C. 1395nn. A financial relationship includes ownership, investment interest, and compensation arrangements. 42 U.S.C. 1395nn(h)(5). The term "referral" is defined more broadly than merely recommending a vendor of DHS to a patient. Instead, the term "referral" means, for Medicare Part B services, "the request by a physician for the item or service" and, for all other services, "the request or establishment of a plan of care by a physician which includes the provision of the designated health service." DHS includes clinical laboratory services as well as the following: physical-therapy services; occupational-therapy services; radiology, including magnetic resonance imaging, computerized axial tomography scans, and ultrasound services; radiation-therapy services and supplies; durable medical equipment and supplies; parenteral and enteral nutrients, equipment, and supplies; prosthetics, orthotics, and prosthetic devices; home health services and supplies; outpatient prescription drugs; and inpatient and outpatient hospital services. The Stark Law contains several exceptions. They include physician services, in-office ancillary services, ownership in publicly traded securities and mutual funds, rental of office space and equipment, bona fide employment relationship, etc. The law is named for United States Congressman Pete Stark (D-CA) who sponsored the initial bill.

Dual diagnosis: (also called co-occurring disorders, COD) is the condition of suffering from a mental illness and a co morbid substance abuse problem. There is considerable debate surrounding the appropriateness of using a single category for a heterogeneous group of individuals with complex needs and a varied range of problems. The concept can be used broadly, for example, depression and alcoholism, or it can be restricted to specify severe mental illness (e.g. psychosis, schizophrenia) and substance misuse disorder (e.g. cannabis abuse), or a person who has a milder mental illness and a drug dependency, such as panic disorder or generalized anxiety disorder and is dependent on opioids. Diagnosing a primary psychiatric illness in substance abusers is challenging as drug abuse itself often induces psychiatric symptoms, thus making it necessary to differentiate between substance induced and preexisting mental illness. Those with co-occurring disorders face complex challenges. They have increased rates of relapse, hospitalization, homelessness, and HIV and Hepatitis C infection compared to those with either mental or substance use disorders alone. The cause of co-occurring disorders is unknown, although there are several theories.

Marketing: is communicating the value of a product, service or brand to customers, for the purpose of promoting or selling that product, service, or brand. Marketing techniques include choosing target markets through market analysis and market segmentation, as well as understanding consumer behavior and advertising a product's value to the customer. From a societal point of view, marketing is the link between a society's material requirements and its economic patterns of response. Marketing satisfies these needs and wants through exchange processes and building long-term relationships. Marketing blends art and applied science (such as behavioral sciences) and makes use of information technology. Marketing is applied in enterprise and organizations through marketing management.

The Baker Act: The Florida Mental Health Act of 1971 (Florida Statute 394.451-394.47891[1] (2009 rev.)), commonly known as the "Baker Act," allows the involuntary institutionalization and examination of an individual. The Baker Act allows for involuntary examination (what some call emergency or involuntary commitment). It can be initiated by judges, law enforcement officials, physicians, or mental health professionals. There must be evidence that the person: possibly has a mental illness (as defined in the Baker Act). Is a harm to self, harm to others, or self-neglectful (as defined in the Baker Act)? Examinations may last up to seventy-two hours after a person is deemed medically stable and occur in over 100 Florida Department of Children and Families-designated receiving facilities statewide. There are many possible outcomes following examination of the patient. This includes the release of the individual to the community (or other community placement), a petition for involuntary inpatient placement (what some call civil commitment), involuntary outpatient placement (what some call outpatient commitment or assisted treatment orders), or voluntary treatment (if the person is competent to consent to voluntary treatment and consents to voluntary treatment). The involuntary outpatient placement language in the Baker Act took effect as part of the Baker Act reform in 2005. The act was named for a Florida state representative from Miami, Maxine Baker, who had a strong interest in mental health issues, served as chair of a House Committee on Mental Health, and was the sponsor of the bill.

What is the Marchman Act?

The Hal S. Marchman Alcohol and Other Drug Services Act of 1993, or more commonly referred to as the Marchman Act, provides for emergency assistance and temporary detention for individual requiring substance abuse evaluation and treatment in the state of Florida. When properly applied to a well-balanced, long-term plan, the Marchman Act has the potential to help an individual reach a healthy bottom by putting into place a court-ordered framework to help support their recovery.

How does the Marchman Act Work?

The Marchman Act is initiated by filing a petition for involuntary assessment in the county court where the impaired individual resides. The petition must be filed in good faith by a person recognized by the court to do so. The petitioner must have reason to believe, and/or direct knowledge that an individual has lost the power of self-control with regard to substance abuse and that there exists the likelihood that the individual has the potential to inflict harm upon themselves or others unless they get help. Furthermore, it must also be demonstrated that the impaired individual is without the capacity to make rational decisions with regard to appreciating the need for treatment. Once all relevant testimony has been heard by the court, it may enter an order for involuntary assessment to assess and stabilize the impaired individual for a period not to exceed five days. The findings of that assessment are then reviewed with the court, which may then enter an order for involuntary treatment for a period not to exceed sixty days. Keeping those proceedings in mind, in the hands of a well-trained professional interventionist, working with the support of like-minded professionals within the legal community, the Marchman Act can be introduced by the friends and family of the impaired individual as a healthy boundary to actually help them break through their own level of resistance.

Integrity: is a concept of consistency of actions, values, methods, measures, principles, expectations, and outcomes. Barbara Killinger offers a traditional definition: Integrity is a personal choice, an uncompromising and predictably consistent commitment to honor moral, ethical, spiritual and artistic values and principles. In ethics, integrity is regarded as the honesty and truthfulness or accuracy of one's actions. Integrity can stand in opposition to hypocrisy, in that judging with the standards of integrity involves regarding internal consistency as a virtue, and suggests that parties holding within themselves apparently conflicting values should account for the discrepancy or alter their beliefs.

The word integrity evolved from the Latin adjective integer, meaning whole or complete. In this context, integrity is the inner sense of "wholeness" deriving from qualities such as honesty and consistency of character. As such, one may judge that others "have integrity" to the extent that they act according to the values, beliefs, and principles they claim to hold.

A value system's abstraction depth and range of applicable interaction may also function as significant factors in identifying integrity due to their congruence or lack of congruence with observation. A value system may evolve over time while retaining integrity if those who espouse the values account for and resolve inconsistencies.

In discussions on behavior and morality, an individual is said to possess the virtue of integrity if the individual's actions are based upon an internally consistent framework of principles. These principles should uniformly adhere to sound logical axioms or postulates. One can describe a person as having ethical integrity to the extent that the individual's actions, beliefs, methods, measures, and principles all derive from a single core group of values. An individual must, therefore, be flexible and willing to adjust these values in order to maintain consistency when these values are challenged; such as when an expected test result fails to be congruent with all observed outcomes. Because such flexibility is a form of accountability, it is regarded as a moral responsibility as well as a virtue.

An individual's value system provides a framework within which the individual acts in ways, which are consistent and expected. Integrity can be seen as the state or condition of having such a framework and acting congruently within the given framework.

One essential aspect of a consistent framework is its avoidance of any unwarranted (arbitrary) exceptions for a particular person or group — especially the person or group that holds the framework. In law, this principle of universal application requires that even those in positions of official power be subject to the same laws as pertain to their fellow citizens. In personal ethics, this principle requires that one should not act according to any rule that one would not wish to see universally followed. For example, one should not steal unless one would want to live in a world in which everyone was a thief. The philosopher Immanuel Kant formally described the principle of universal application in his categorical imperative.

The concept of integrity implies wholeness, a comprehensive corpus of beliefs often referred to as a worldview. This concept of wholeness emphasizes honesty and authenticity, requiring that one act at all times in accordance with the individual's chosen worldview. Ayn Rand considered that integrity "does not consist of loyalty to one's subjective whims, but of loyalty to rational principles". Ethical integrity is not synonymous with the good, as Zuckert and Zuckert show about Ted Bundy: When caught, he defended his actions in terms of the fact-value distinction. He scoffed at those, like the professors from whom he learned the fact-value distinction, who still lived their lives as if there were truth-value to value claims. He thought they were fools and that he was one of the few who had the courage and integrity to live a consistent life in light of the truth that value judgments, including the command "Thou shall not kill," are merely subjective assertions. —Zuckert and Zuckert, The truth about Leo Strauss: political philosophy and American democracy

Informed Consent: is a process for getting permission before conducting a healthcare intervention on a person. A health care provider may ask a patient to consent to receive therapy before providing it, or a clinical researcher may ask a research participant before enrolling that person into a clinical trial. Informed consent is collected according to guidelines from the fields of medical ethics and research ethics. An informed consent can be said to have been given based upon a clear appreciation and understanding of the facts, implications, and future consequences of an action. In order to give informed consent, the individual concerned must have adequate reasoning faculties and be in possession of all relevant facts at the time consent is given. Impairments to reasoning and judgment which may make it impossible for someone to give informed consent include such factors as basic intellectual or emotional immaturity, high levels of stress such as PTSD or a severe intellectual disability, severe mental illness, intoxication, severe sleep deprivation, Alzheimer's disease, or being in a coma.

Some acts can take place because of a lack of informed consent. In cases where an individual is considered unable to give informed consent, another person is generally authorized to give consent on his behalf, e.g., parents or legal guardians of a child (though in this circumstance the child may be required to provide informed assent) and conservators for the mentally ill. In cases where an individual is provided insufficient information to form a reasoned decision, serious ethical issues arise. Such cases in a clinical trial in medical research are anticipated and prevented by an ethics committee or Institutional Review Board.

Competence (or competency): is the ability of an individual to do a job properly. A competency is a set of defined behaviors that provide a structured guide enabling the identification, evaluation, and development of the behaviors in individual employees. The term "competence" first appeared in an article authored by R.W. White in 1959 as a concept for performance motivation. Later, in 1970, Craig C. Lundberg defined the concept in "Planning the Executive Development Program". The term gained traction when in 1973, David McClelland, Ph.D. wrote a seminal paper entitled, "Testing for Competence Rather Than for Intelligence". It has since been popularized by one-time fellow McBer & Company (Currently the "Hay Group") colleague Richard Boyatzis and many others, such as T.F. Gilbert (1978) who used the concept in relationship to performance improvement. Its use varies widely, which leads to considerable misunderstanding. Some scholars see "competence" as a combination of practical and theoretical knowledge, cognitive skills, behavior, and values used to improve performance; or as the state or quality of being adequately or well qualified, having the ability to perform a specific role. For instance, life, management competency might include systems thinking and emotional intelligence, and skills in influence and negotiation. Competency is also used as a more general description of the requirements of human beings in organizations and communities. Competency is sometimes thought of as being shown in action in a situation and context that might be different the next time a person has to act. In emergencies, competent people may react to a situation following behaviors they have previously found to succeed. To be competent a person would need to be able to interpret the situation in the context and to have a repertoire of possible actions to take and have trained in the possible actions in the repertoire if this is relevant. Regardless of training, competency would grow through experience and the extent of an individual to learn and adapt. Competency has different meanings and continues to remain one of the most diffuse terms in the management development sector and the organizational and occupational literature. Competencies are also what people need to be successful in their jobs. Job competencies are not the same as job task. Competencies include all the related knowledge, skills, abilities, and attributes that form a person's job. This set of context-specific qualities is correlated with superior job performance and can be used as a standard against which to measure job performance as well as to develop, recruit, and hire employees. Competencies and competency models may be applicable to all employees in an organization or they may be position specific. Identifying employee competencies can contribute to improved organizational performance. They are most effective if they meet several critical standards, including linkage to, and leverage within an organization's human resource system Core competencies differentiate an organization from its competition and create a company's competitive advantage in the marketplace. An organizational core competency is its strategic strength. Competencies provide organizations with a way to define in behavioral terms what it is that people need to do to produce the results that the organization desires, in a way that is keeping with its culture. By having competencies defined in the organization, it allows employees to know what they need to be productive. When properly defined, competencies, allows organizations to evaluate the extent to which behaviors employees are demonstrating and where they may be lacking. For competencies where employees are lacking, they can learn. This will allow organizations to know potentially what resources they may need to help the employee develop and learn those competencies. Competencies can distinguish and differentiate your organization from your competitors. While two organizations may be alike in financial results, the way in which the results were achieve could be different based on the competencies that fit their particular strategy and organizational culture. Lastly, competencies can provide a structured model that can be used to integrate management practices throughout the organization. Competencies that align their recruiting, performance management, training and development and reward practices to reinforce key behaviors that the organization values.

Ethics: sometimes known as philosophical ethics, ethical theory, moral theory, and moral philosophy, is a branch of philosophy that involves systematizing, defending and recommending concepts of right and wrong conduct, often addressing disputes of moral diversity. The term comes from the Greek word ἠθικός ethikos from ἦθος ethos, which means "custom, habit". The super field within philosophy known as axiology includes both ethics and aesthetics and is unified by each sub-branch's concern with value. Philosophical ethics investigates what is the best way for humans to live, and what kinds of actions are right or wrong circumstances. Ethics may be divided into three major areas of study:

- Meta-ethics, about the theoretical meaning and reference of moral propositions and how their truth values (if any) may be determined
- Normative ethics, about the practical means of determining a moral course of action
- Applied ethics draws upon ethical theory in order to ask what a person is obligated to do in some very specific situation, or within some domain of action (such as business)

Related fields are moral psychology, descriptive ethics, and value theory. Ethics seeks to resolve questions dealing with human morality—concepts such as good and evil, right and wrong, virtue and vice, justice and crime. Richard Paul and Linda Elder of the Foundation for Critical Thinking define ethics as "a set of concepts and principles that guide us in determining what behavior helps or harms sentient creatures". The Cambridge Dictionary of Philosophy states that the word ethics is "commonly used interchangeably with 'morality' ... and sometimes it is used more narrowly to mean the moral principles of a particular tradition, group or individual." Paul and Elder state that, "most people confuse ethics with behaving in accordance with social conventions, religious beliefs and the law", and don't treat ethics as a stand-alone concept. The word ethics in English can mean several things. It can refer to philosophical ethics—a project that attempts to use reason in order to answer various kinds of ethical questions. It can also be used to describe a particular person's own, idiosyncratic principles or habits. For example: "Joe has good ethics." It may also be used to characterize the questions of right-conduct in some specific sphere, even when such right-conduct is not examined philosophically: "business ethics," or "the ethics of child-rearing" may refer, but need not refer, to a philosophical examination of such issues. Philosophical ethics, or "ethical theory," is not the exclusive use of the term "ethics" in English.

Standards: A standards organization, standards body, standards developing organization (SDO), or standards setting organization (SSO) is any organization whose primary activities are developing, coordinating, promulgating, revising, amending, reissuing, interpreting, or otherwise producing technical standards that are intended to address the needs of some relatively wide base of affected adopters. Most standards are voluntary in the sense that they are offered for adoption by people or industry without being mandated in law. Some standards become mandatory when they are adopted by regulators as legal requirements in particular domains. The term formal standard refers specifically to a specification that has been approved by a standards setting organization. The term de jure standard refers to a standard mandated by legal requirements or refers generally to any formal standard. In contrast, the term de facto standard refers to a specification (or protocol or technology) that has achieved widespread use and acceptance – often without being approved by any standards organization (or receiving such approval only after it already has achieved widespread use). Examples of de facto standards that were not approved by any standards organizations (or at least not approved until after they were in widespread de facto use) include the Hayes command set developed by Hayes, Apple's TrueType font design and the PCL protocol used by Hewlett-Packard in the computer printers they produced.

Normally, the term standards organization is not used to refer to the individual parties participating within the standards developing organization in the capacity of founders, benefactors, stakeholders, members or contributors, who themselves may function as the standards organizations.

A principle: is a law or rule that has to be, or usually is to be followed, or can be desirably followed, or is an inevitable consequence of something, such as the laws observed in nature or the way that a system is constructed. The principles of such a system are understood by its users as the essential characteristics of the system, or reflecting system's designed purpose, and the effective operation or use of which would be impossible if any one of the principles was to be ignored.

Examples of principles:

- Descriptive comprehensive and fundamental law, doctrine, or assumption
- Normative rule or code of conduct
- Law or fact of nature underlying the working of an artificial device

Quality: in business, engineering and manufacturing has a pragmatic interpretation as the non-inferiority or superiority of something; it is also defined as fitness for purpose. Quality is a perceptual, conditional, and somewhat subjective attribute and may be understood differently by different people. Consumers may focus on the specification quality of a product/service, or how it compares to competitors in the marketplace. Producers might measure the conformance quality, or degree to which the product/service was produced correctly. Support personnel may measure quality in the degree that a product is reliable, maintainable, or sustainable. Simply put, a quality item (an item that has quality) has the ability to perform satisfactorily in service and is suitable for its intended purpose.

There are five aspects of quality in a business context:

1. Producing – providing something.
2. Checking – confirming that something has been done correctly.
3. Quality Control – controlling a process to ensure that the outcomes are predictable.
4. Quality Management – directing an organization so that it optimizes its performance through analysis and improvement.
5. Quality Assurance – obtaining confidence that a product or service will be satisfactory. (Normally performed by a purchaser)

Quality applied in these forms was mainly developed by the procurement directorates of NASA, the military, and nuclear industries from the 1960s and this is why so much emphasis was placed on Quality Assurance. The original versions of Quality Management System Standards (eventually merged to ISO 9001) were designed to contract manufacturers to produce better products, consistently and were focused on Producing, Checking, and Quality Control.

The subsequent move of the Quality sector toward management systems can be clearly seen by the aggregation of the product quality requirements into one-eighth of the current version of ISO 9001. This increased focus on Quality Management has promoted a general perception that quality is about procedures and documentation. Similar experiences can be seen in the areas of Safety Management Systems and Environmental Management Systems.

The emergence of tools like Asset Optimization and six sigma is an interesting development in the application of quality principles in business.

Managing quality is fundamental to any activity and having a clear understanding of the five aspects, measuring performance and taking action to improve is essential to an organizations survival and growth.

Respect: is a positive feeling of esteem or deference for a person or other entity (such as a nation or a religion), and also specific actions and conduct representative of that esteem. Respect can be a specific feeling of regard for the actual qualities of the one respected (e.g., "I have great respect for her judgment"). It can also be conducted in accord with a specific ethic of respect. Rude conduct is usually considered to indicate a lack of respect, disrespect, whereas actions that honor somebody or something indicate respect. Specific ethics of respect are of fundamental importance to various cultures. Respect for tradition and legitimate authority is identified by Jonathan Haidt, a professor at the New York University Stern School of Business, as one of five fundamental moral values shared to a greater or lesser degree by different societies and individuals. Respect can be both given and/or received. Depending on an individual's cultural reference frame, respect can be something that is earned. Respect is often thought of as earned or built over time. Often, continued caring interactions are required to maintain or increase feelings of respect among individuals. Chivalry, by some definitions, contains the outward display of respect. Respect should not be confused with tolerance. The antonym and opposite of respect is disrespect. For others in society, some people earn the respect of individuals by assisting others or playing important social roles. In many cultures, individuals are considered to be worthy of respect until they prove otherwise. Courtesies that show respect include simple words and phrases like "thank you" in the West, simple physical gestures like a slight bow in the East, a smile or direct eye contact. A woman's masculinity in East Asia may make it more difficult for her to gain respect in the workplace. In the book the sexual intercourse, Stevi Jackson, Liu Jieyu, and Woo Juhyun state, "Women had to make a double effort to maintain their aesthetic self-image. When presenting themselves in the work environment, they had gone through careful management of gender display." This wall makes it difficult in the work place as respect, in that environment, is based on the reality of skill and personality, not on an assumption of proper behavior. Chinese women are placed in a situation in the workplace that creates a great compromise. They are expected to exhibit a more open sexuality than what is normally accepted in the social environment, but at the same time are being very sexually entertained. Hiroko Hayashi, states in his article, Sexual Harassment in the Workplace and Equal Employment Legislation, that more recently the total number of female Japanese workers has increased, which has been accompanied by a major development in sexual harassment as a form of sexual employment discrimination. "In Japan, sexual harassment has been defined as "unwelcome remarks and conduct in the workplace which influence a worker's job performance and cause a hostile work environment." In the Fukuoka District Court on April 16, 1992, the first Japanese case for, "Seiteki Iyagarese" or "sexual unpleasantness" in the workplace was seen as a violation of a worker's interest in maintaining the honor of her reputation. Some women decide to abstain from the social environment to keep their respect. Men can also be sexually harassed in the workplace. During the Economic Times-Synovate survey in India, it was found that out of 527 people, across seven cities, 19% of men have faced sexual harassment at the workplace.

A professional: is a member of a profession. The term also describes the standards of education and training that prepare members of the profession with the knowledge and skills necessary to perform the role of that profession. In addition, most professionals are subject to strict codes of conduct enshrining rigorous ethical and moral obligations. Professional standards of practice and ethics for a particular field are typically agreed upon and maintained through widely recognized professional associations. Some definitions of "professional" limit this term to those professions that serve some important aspect of public interest and the general good of society. In some cultures, the term is used as shorthand to describe a particular social stratum of well-educated workers who enjoy considerable work autonomy and who are commonly engaged in creative and intellectually challenging work.

Legal Governance, Risk Management, and Compliance or "LGRC": refers to the complex set of processes, rules, tools, and systems used by corporate legal departments to adopt, implement and monitor an integrated approach to business problems. While Governance, Risk Management, and Compliance refers to a generalized set of tools for managing a corporation or company, Legal GRC, or LGRC, refers to a specialized – but similar – set of tools utilized by attorneys, corporate legal departments, general counsel and law firms to govern themselves and their corporations, especially but not exclusively in relation to the law. Other specializations within the realm of governance, risk management, and compliance include IT GRC and financial GRC. Within these three realms, there is a great deal of overlap, particularly in large corporations that have legal and IT departments, as well as financial departments. Legal risk management refers to the process of evaluating alternative regulatory and non-regulatory responses to risk and selecting among them. Even with the legal realm, this process requires knowledge of the legal, economic, and social factors, as well as knowledge of the business world in which legal teams operate. In an organizational setting, risk management refers to the process, by which an organization sets the risk tolerance, identifies potential risks and prioritizes the tolerance for risk based on the organization's business objectives, and manages and mitigates risks throughout the organization.

Legal compliance: is the process or procedure to ensure that an organization follows relevant laws, regulations, and business rules. The definition of legal compliance, especially in the context of corporate legal departments, has recently been expanded to include understanding and adhering to ethical codes within entire professions, as well. There are two requirements for an enterprise to be compliant with the law, first, its policies need to be consistent with the law. Second, its policies need to be complete with respect to the law. The role of legal compliance has also been expanded to include self-monitoring the non-governed behavior with industries and corporations that could lead to workplace indiscretions. Within the LGRC realm, it is important to keep in mind that if a strong legal governance component is in place, risk can be accurately assessed and the monitoring of legal compliance be carried out efficiently. It is also important to realize that within the LGRC framework, legal teams work closely with executive teams and other business departments to align their goals and ensure proper communication.

Mandatory Reporting: In many jurisdictions, such as US, Canada, much of Europe and Australia, mandated reporters are people who have regular contact with vulnerable people such as children, disabled persons and senior citizens and are therefore legally required to report (or cause a report to be made) when abuse is observed or suspected. Specific details vary between jurisdictions- the abuse that must be reported may include financial, physical, sexual, neglect, or other types of abuse. Mandated reporters may include paid or unpaid people who have assumed full or intermittent responsibility for the care of a child, dependent adult, or elder. History of mandatory reporting. In 1962, two doctors (Henry Kempe and Brandt Steele) published "The Battered Child Syndrome" which helped doctors identify child abuse, its effects, and the need to report serious physical abuse (i.e. fractures) to legal authorities. In 1974, the US Congress passed the Child Abuse Prevention and Treatment Act (CAPTA), with funds to states for development of Child Protective Services (CPS) and hotlines to prevent serious injuries to children. These laws and the accompanying media campaigns, research, conferences, trainings, books/journal articles brought about a gradual change in societal expectations on reporting in the US and, at different rates in other western nations.

Although originally the focus was on serious physical abuse in the US, it slowly evolved to include sexual and emotional abuse and neglect, including bruising, developmental delay, psychological harm, and exposure to domestic abuse in many countries, primarily in Northern America, Europe, and Australia/ New Zealand. In the US, there was a 2348% increase in hotline calls from 150,000 in 1963 to 3.3 million in 2009. In 2011, there were 3.4 million calls. From 1992 to 2009 in the US, substantiated cases of sexual abuse declined 62%, physical abuse decreased 56% and neglect 10%. Although the referrals increase each year, about 1% of the child population is affected by any form of substantiated maltreatment. Referrals increase each year, but the actual substantiated cases remain low and are approximately the same or decline each year. Overall, the total number of substantiations in Australia has nearly doubled since 2001 (1.77 times higher) but have shown a slight downward trend since 2005-06. Specific comparisons cannot be made before this time, as different jurisdictions have made substantial changes throughout this period in reporting requirements and definitions of terms.

Self-disclosure: is a process of communication through which one person reveals himself or herself to another. It comprises everything an individual chooses to tell the other person about himself or herself, making him or her known. The information can be descriptive or evaluative and can include thoughts, feelings, aspirations, goals, failures, successes, fears, dreams as well as one's likes, dislikes, and favorites. According to social penetration theory, there are two dimensions to self-disclosure: breadth and depth. Both are crucial in developing a fully intimate relationship. The range of topics discussed by two individuals is the breadth of disclosure. The degree to which the information revealed is private or personal is the depth of that disclosure. It is easier for breadth to be expanded first in a relationship because of its more accessible features; it consists of outer layers of personality and everyday lives, such as occupations and preferences. Depth is more difficult to reach, given its inner location; it includes painful memories and more unusual traits that we might try to hide from most people. This is why we reveal ourselves most thoroughly and discuss the widest range of topics with our spouses and loved ones.

Self-disclosure is an important building block for intimacy; intimacy cannot be achieved without it. We expect self-disclosure to be reciprocal and appropriate. Self-disclosure can be assessed by an analysis of cost and rewards, which can be further explained by social exchange theory. Most self-disclosure occurs early in relational development, but more intimate self-disclosure occurs later. The Employment Non-Discrimination Act (ENDA): is legislation proposed in the United States Congress that would prohibit discrimination in hiring and employment on the basis of sexual orientation or gender identity by employers with at least fifteen employees. ENDA has been introduced in every Congress since 1994 except the 109th. Similar legislation has been introduced without passage since 1974. The bill gained its best chance at passing after the Democratic Party broke twelve years of Republican Congressional rule in the 2006 midterm elections. In 2007, gender identity protections were added to the legislation for the first time. Some sponsors believed that even with a Democratic majority, ENDA did not have enough votes to pass the House of Representatives with transgender inclusion and dropped it from the bill, which passed the House and then died in the Senate. President George W. Bush threatened to veto the measure. LGBT advocacy organizations and the LGBT community were divided over support of the modified bill. In 2009, following Democratic gains in the 2008, elections, and after the divisiveness of the 2007 debate, Rep. Barney Frank introduced a transgender-inclusive version of ENDA. He introduced it again in 2011, and Sen. Jeff Merkley introduced it in the Senate. On November 7, 2013, Merkley's bill passed the Senate with bipartisan support by a vote of 64-32. President Barack Obama supports the bill's passage. Communication privacy management theory, originally known as communication boundary management: is a communication theory first developed by Sandra Petronio. Petronio's conclusions are relevant to the study of communication because before Communication Boundary Management there was only one other theory that studied self-disclosure, Social Penetration Theory. While both communication privacy management theory and social penetration theory are based in self-disclosure, the critical difference is that CPM focuses on understanding "the conceptual idea of disclosure". Communication Privacy Management theory describes the ways in which relational actors manage their privacy boundaries and the disclosure of private information. The theory focuses heavily on the processes that people employ to determine when and how they choose to conceal or reveal private information. Through this theory, Petronio describes the ever-present dialectic of privacy and openness within various relationship models, explains how relationships develop as public and private boundaries are negotiated and coordinated, and demonstrates how individuals regulate revealing and concealing information through communication.

Harm Prevention: When you hire better employees than your competitor, you are at a distinct advantage. The ability to keep those employees healthy and productive is critical in propelling your business to a higher and more efficient arena.

Providing services that promote health and wellness in the workplace, from prework screening to injury prevention, decreases worker's compensation costs and promotes a culture of caring, safety, and good business practice. Primum non nocere is a Latin phrase that means "first, do no harm." The phrase is sometimes recorded as primum nil nocere.

Non-malfeasance, which is derived from the maxim, is one of the principal precepts of bioethics that all healthcare students are taught in school and is a fundamental principle throughout the world. Another way to state it is that, "given an existing problem, it may be better not to do something, or even to do nothing, than to risk causing more harm than good." It reminds the health care provider that they must consider the possible harm that any intervention might do. It is invoked when debating the use of an intervention that carries an obvious risk of harm but a less certain chance of benefit.

Non-malfeasance is often contrasted with its corollary, beneficence.

A conflict of interest (COI): is a situation occurring when an individual or organization is involved in multiple interests, one of which could possibly corrupt the motivation.

The presence of a conflict of interest is independent of the occurrence of impropriety. Therefore, a conflict of interest can be discovered and voluntarily defused before any corruption occurs. A widely used definition is: "A conflict of interest is a set of circumstances that creates a risk that professional judgment or actions regarding a primary interest will be unduly influenced by a secondary interest." Primary interest refers to the principal goals of the profession or activity, such as the protection of clients, the health of patients, the integrity of research, and the duties of public office. Secondary interest includes not only financial gain but also such motives as the desire for professional advancement and the wish to do favors for family and friends, but conflict of interest rules usually focus on financial relationships because they are relatively more objective, fungible, and quantifiable. The secondary interests are not treated as wrong in themselves but become objectionable when they are believed to have greater weight than the primary interests. The conflict in a conflict of interest exists whether or not an individual is influenced by the secondary interest. It exists if the circumstances are reasonably believed (on the basis of experience and objective evidence) to create a risk that decisions may be unduly influenced by secondary interests.

Confidentiality: is commonly applied to conversations between doctors and patients. Legal protections prevent physicians from revealing certain discussions with patients, even under oath in court. This physician-patient privilege only applies to secrets shared between physician and patient during the course of providing medical care.

The rule dates back to at least the Hippocratic Oath, which reads: Whatever, in connection with my professional service, or not in connection with it, I see or hear, in the life of men, which ought not to be spoken of abroad, I will not divulge, as reckoning that all such should be kept secret.

Traditionally, medical ethics has viewed the duty of confidentiality as a relatively nonnegotiable tenet of medical practice.

Confidentiality: is mandated in America by HIPAA laws, specifically the Privacy Rule, and various state laws, some more rigorous than HIPAA. However, numerous exceptions to the rules have been carved out over the years. For example, many American states require physicians to report gunshot wounds to the police and impaired drivers to the Department of Motor Vehicles. Confidentiality is also challenged in cases involving the diagnosis of a sexually transmitted disease in a patient who refuses to reveal the diagnosis to a spouse, and in the termination of a pregnancy in an underage patient, without the knowledge of the patient's parents. Many states in the US have laws governing parental notification in underage abortion. Clinical and counseling psychology: The ethical principle of confidentiality requires that information shared by the client with the therapist in the course of treatment is not shared with others. This is important for the therapeutic alliance, as it promotes an environment of trust. There are important exceptions to confidentiality, namely where it conflicts with the clinician's duty to warn or duty to protect. This includes instances of suicidal behavior or homicidal plans, child abuse, elder abuse and dependent adult abuse. On 26 June 2012, a judge of Oslo District Court apologized for the court's hearing of testimony (on 14 June, regarding contact with Child Welfare Services (Norway)) that was covered by confidentiality (that had not been waived at that point of the trial of Anders Behring Breivik).

(Information & Definitions from Wikipedia)

Rev. Dr. Kevin T. Coughlin Ph.D. Publication Credits

KTC Publishing Phase IIC Coaching, LLC Amazon.com *The Official Gambling Addiction Recovery Coach's Workbook* 2017

KTC Publishing Phase IIC Coaching, LLC Amazon.com *The Official Gambling Addiction Christian Recovery Coach's Workbook* 2017

KTC Publishing Phase IIC Coaching, LLC Amazon.com *My Daily Pet Journal Book; I Love Cats* 2017

KTC Publishing Phase IIC Coaching, LLC Amazon.com *My Daily Pet Journal Book; I Love Dogs* 2017

KTC Publishing Phase IIC Coaching, LLC Amazon.com *Christian Coaching; Life Recovery Coaching Workbook and Journal 2017* Made the Amazon Top 100 Best-Seller List

KTC Publishing Phase IIC Coaching, LLC Amazon.com **Christian Coaching: The Master's Guide to Becoming a Professional Christian Life and Recovery Coach** 2017 Made the Amazon.com Top 100 Best-Seller list

KTC Publishing Phase IIC Coaching, LLC Amazon.com *Addiction Professionals AMA/ APA Guide.* 2017 Made the Amazon.com Top 100 Best-Seller list

KTC Publishing Phase IIC Coaching, LLC Amazon.com *My Monthly Journal; A Roadmap for Change.* 2017 Made the Amazon.com Top 100 Best-Seller list

KTC Publishing Phase IIC Coaching, LLC Amazon.com *My Daily Food Journal; A Daily Food Action Plan for Success.* 2017 Made the Amazon.com Top 100 Best-Seller list

KTC Publishing Phase IIC Coaching, LLC Amazon.com *My Daily Prayer Journal; A Walk with Jesus.* 2017 Made the Amazon.com Top 100 Best-Seller list

KTC Publishing Phase IIC Coaching, LLC Amazon.com *My Monthly Journal Book; a Roadmap for Success.* 2017 Made the Amazon.com Top 100 Best-Seller list

KTC Publishing Phase IIC Coaching, LLC Amazon.com *My Daily Meditation Book.* 2017 Made the Amazon.com Top 100 Best-Seller list

KTC Publishing Phase IIC Coaching, LLC Amazon.com *We Can the Anthology; A Collection of Poetry, A Journey Through Addiction and Recovery* 2017

KTC Publishing Phase IIC Coaching, LLC Amazon.com *Prevention; Teaching Teens to Say No to Drugs.* 2017 Made the Amazon.com Top 100 Best-Seller list.

KTC Publishing Phase IIC Coaching, LLC Amazon.com *Relapse Prevention; Long-Term Sobriety.* 2017 Made the Amazon.com Top 100 Best-Seller list.

KTC Publishing Phase IIC Coaching, LLC Amazon.com *Thirty Days of Thoughts About the Holidays.* 2016 Made the Amazon.com Top 100 Best-Seller list.

KTC Publishing Phase IIC Coaching, LLC Amazon.com *Thirty Days of Thoughts About Christian Recovery and the Holidays.* 2016 Made the Amazon.com Top 100 Best-Seller list.

KTC Publishing Phase IIC Coaching, LLC Amazon.com *Recovery & Life Coaching; The Official Workbook for Coaches and Their Clients*. Co-Author Dr. Cali Estes 2016 #1 Best-Seller Amazon.com Top 100 Best-Seller List

KTC Publishing Phase IIC Coaching, LLC Amazon.com *Addictions: What All Parents Need to Know to Survive the Drug Epidemic.* 2016 Made the Amazon.com Top 100 Best-Seller list.

KTC Publishing Phase IIC Coaching, LLC Amazon.com If You Want What We Have; A Journey Through the Twelve Steps of Recovery Workbook and Manual 2015 Made the Amazon.com Top 100 Best-Seller list.

KTC Publishing Phase IIC Coaching, LLC Amazon.com *In the Sunlight of the Spirit* Workbook and Manual 2015

KTC Publishing Phase IIC Coaching, LLC Amazon.com *We Can; A Collection of Poetry, A Journey Through Addiction and Recovery 2016*

KTC Publishing Phase IIC Coaching, LLC Amazon.com *We Can 2; A Collection of Poetry, A Journey Through Addiction and Recovery 2016*

KTC Publishing Phase IIC Coaching, LLC Amazon.com *We Can 3; A Collection of Poetry, A Journey Through Addiction and Recovery 2016*

Tumbleweeds; Feather Books Poetry Series a Book of Poetry Written by Rev. Kevin T. Coughlin Feather Books England May 2002 (In Memory of DeWitt)

Wayne Independent Newspaper Honesdale, PA

News Eagle, Hawley, PA

Reading Eagle, Reading, PA Berks & Beyond

www.addictsrehab.com

My RecoveryRadio.com Host Kent Paul Sept. 11[Th], 2016 Interview

BBS Radio Poetry reading

Blog Talk Radio - Interviews

The Serenity Show - Interview

Passion Diva Radio- Interview

Recovery Starts Here- Interview

www.sacredearthpartners.com - Interview

The Broken Brain (Blog Talk Radio) - Interview

www.eatingdisorderhope.com

Keys to Recovery Newspaper Beth Dewey CEO

www.keystorecovery.com

All 4 Ur Addiction Recovery Referral Resource Guide Jenny Clark Owner

Tripadvisor.com

MindBodyNetwork

Grieving Behind the Badge Peggy Sweeny Founder

www.theaddictsmom.com

In Recovery Magazine

The Sober World Magazine

The Soberworld.com

Shout My Book

Bookgoodies.com

Goodreads

Book Reader Magazine

Awesomegang.com

www.christiancoaches.com

Hardrock Favorites

Metalcorp

SixxAMFansPhotos

NEWS CHANNEL 10 EYEWITNESS NEWS CHANNEL.COM
KHQQ6 ABC NEWS
ABC EYEWITNESS NEWS 8 KLKN-TV
FOX14 NEWS AT 9
Erie News Now
NTV Nebraska.TV ABC
Western Mass News Channels 3 ABC 40 Fox 6
ABC9 KTRE
7 KLTV ABC
Fox 19 Now
KXNEWC Eyewitness News
12 WSFA ABC
ABC 6 News WLNE TV
100.7 KFM BFM
Fox 5 KVVU-TV Local Los Vegas
13 WTHR COM Indians News ABC
Eyewitness News 3 WFSB.COM
Fox 12 Oregon
WDRB.COM
Fox29 WFFX.COM
WETV San Diego
HAWAII News Now
Marketers Media
WALB News 10 ABC
Tristate Update.com 13 News WOWK
AM760
WMBF ABC News
KCEN HD ABC KCENTV.COM
WECT6 ABC News
Eyewitness News3 WFSB.COM
WLOX ABC BOUNCE Eyewitness News
Eyewitness News 8
CBS8.COM
News channel 6 KAUZ
SPROUT News
12 Eyewitness News KFVS
KEYC MANKATO News 12 CBS & FOX LOCAL NEWS
3 WRCB TV ABC COM
KNDO 23 NBC
KNDU 25 NBC
RecoveryView.com
The Aurorean, Encircle Publications 1998 Poetry and Essays

Joel's House Publications 1998-2005 Poetry and Essays
Our Journey 1998-2005 Poetry
The Poetry Explosion, The Pen 1999-2003 Poetry
Apostrophe 1998 Poetry
Nuthouse Twin Rivers Press 1998 Poetry
The National Library of Poetry 1998
Lines N' Rhymes 1998 Poetry
The Poetry Church Feather Books
England. Anthology John Hunt Publications 1999 Poetry
A Tapestry in Time. 1999 Poetry Book 18 Poems
Connecticut Department of Mental Health and Addiction Services
The Webster Times 1999 Poetry
The Angel News 1999 Poetry
The Skater won The Editor's Choice Award September 1999 (Our Journey)
The Blind Man's Rainbow 1999 Poetry
Arnazella 2001 Poetry
Feather Books, The Poetry Church 1998-2002
The American Dissident 2002 Poetry
The Good Shepherd Poetry 2002
Ya ' Sou Magazine Essays and Poetry
Colt. Winner Editor's Choice Award Contest Literally Horses 2002
Goodbye My Friend Read on the Radio Rhyme and Reason UBC Europe & the UK September 2001 Read on the Radio in Europe and the UK as a Tribute to those lost on September 11th bombings. My poem was read over the radio for many days.
Tumbleweed Read on BBC Radio in England 2001
Published by Feather Books
Notified by John Waddington Feather that Tumbleweed had been read on BBC Radio in England on Several Occasions.
Stanwich Congregational Flyer Poetry
University of Scranton Aniska College of Professionals Essay 2002
Scranton University 2002 Poetry
The River Reporter Newspaper 2002 Poetry
Unity Community News 2002 Poetry
The Poetry Corner Angelfire.com Poetry
The Poet's Market 2002 Poetry
The Poetry Church England 2003 Poetry
Cover of Wayne Independent News 2003 Poetry
Nomad's Choir 2003 Poetry
Written a series of 9 course manuals for a coaching recovery curriculum. 2014-2015
www.addictedminds.org 2015-2016 Articles
www.soberservices.com 2015 Articles
http://fromaddict2advocate.blogspot 2016 Articles Marilyn Davis

LinkedIn 2014-2016 Articles
Two Drops of Ink S.W. Biddulph 2015- 2016 Poetry/ Articles
The Addict's Mom 2016 Articles Blog
Ghostwriter Articles/ Content 2014-2016
KEITV12: The Kingdom Hour- Interview
BlogTalkRadio The Kingdom Hour- Interview
RecoveryView.com Online Journal Interview
Brooklyn TV Interview
CCE Christian Children's Empowerment

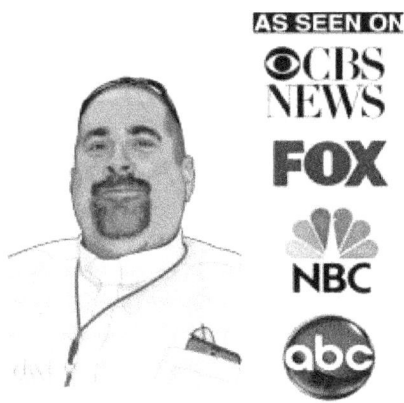

About the Author

Rev. Dr., Kevin T. Coughlin Ph.D., DCC, DDV, DD, IMAC, NCIP is an International Master Coach, trainer, #1 best-selling author, writer, poet, speaker, a Diplomate Christian counselor, and therapist, he is Board Certified in Family, Developmental, Alcoholism, Substance Abuse, and Grief Counseling, the Reverend is a NCIP interventionist, a Domestic Violence Advocate, Associate Professor for DCU, a Provincial Superintendent (to be consecrated a Bishop in 2018) and so much more; he is an expert in the field of Addiction and Recovery. He was a Founder and Board Member of a Residential Recovery Facility New Beginning Ministry, Inc. and is President and CEO of Phase IIC Coaching, LLC., The former Program Director for a coaching school, and the former Editor in Chief for an online treatment directory and blog. The Reverend has over forty-seven years of experience with the AA program. He has been working in the addiction recovery field for almost two decades, has helped thousands of individuals and their families overcome all types of addictions, substance abuse, alcoholism, process addiction, shame and guilt, relationship and communication problems, anger management, inner healing, self-image, interventions and much more. He is a published author and has published thousands of poems and articles published throughout the United States and other Nations, he has been interviewed on numerous radio talk shows, television, published in magazines, newspapers, books, and online publications; he has been featured on ABC, CBS, FOX, NBC, and the BBC in the UK. Rev. Kev is a former State, National & World-Champion Powerlifter, and still holds several records. He loves to write, read, teach, listen to music, and spend time with people and dogs. His parents are his heroes. The Reverend supports several dog rescues.

Follow Rev. Kev. on Social Media

https://www.goodreads.com/author/show/14874631.Kevin_Coughlin

About.me Link: https://about.me/ktc1961/

http://ilikeebooks.com/if-you-want-what-we-have/

http://awesomegang.com

www.amazon.com/Rev.-Kevin-TCoughlin/e/B01AF6AAAI/ref=ntt_dp_epwbk_0

http://www.barnesandnoble.com/w/addictions-what-all-parents-need-to-know-to-survive-the-drug-epidemic-rev-dr-kevin-t-coughlin-phd/1124049106?ean=9780997700695

http://www.barnesandnoble.com/w/in-the-sunlight-of-the-spirit-rev-dr-kevin-t-coughlin/1124049139?ean=9780997700671

http://www.barnesandnoble.com/w/if-you-want-what-we-have-rev-dr-kevin-t-coughlin/1124049130?ean=9780997700688

http://mybookplace.net/in-the-sunlight-of-the-spirit-a Rev. Dr. Kev's Social Media Accounts

Facebook
Kevin Coughlin:
https://www.facebook.com/profile.php?id=100008449955607
My Group, Resources for those suffering from addiction and their families: https://www.facebook.com/groups/resourcesforthosesufferingfromaddiction/
RevKev The Addiction Expert: https://www.facebook.com/RevKev/?fref=ts

LinkedIn
Rev. Dr. Kevin T. Coughlin PhD
https://www.linkedin.com/in/revkevnetwork

Google+
Kevin Coughlin
https://plus.google.com/112400908736308001821/posts
My Group: The Recovery Community Family and Friends:
https://plus.google.com/communities/113521225141112811207

Pinterest
Kevin Coughlin: https://www.pinterest.com/ktc1961/
My Group Board: Recovery We Can
https://www.pinterest.com/ktc1961/recovery-we-can/

Tumblr
https://www.tumblr.com/blog/revkevsrecoveryworld

Instagram
theaddiction.expert

My Websites:
www.revkevsrecoveryworld.com
theaddiction.expert
theaddiction.guru

Twitter:
1. https://twitter.com/AuthorRevKev
Rev. Kev's Goodreads Link:
-spirituality-training-manual-and-workbook-by-Kevin-Coughlin

Friends of Recovery Readers and Reviewers Book Group on Facebook:

https://www.facebook.com/groups/1667708970205824/

Thank you for reading my work! If you enjoyed my book, would you consider reviewing it on Amazon.com? We would appreciate your help in getting the word out on how helpful this book can be in someone's life. Thank you so much and God bless you! Phil 4:13